YOU ARE
SPECIAL TOO

Books in the same series

A Special Book About Me
A Book for Children Diagnosed with Asperger Syndrome
Josie Santomauro
Illustrated by Carla Marino
ISBN 978 1 84310 655 5
Asperger Syndrome: After the Diagnosis series

Mothering Your Special Child
A Book for Mothers or Carers of Children Diagnosed with Asperger Syndrome
Josie Santomauro
Illustrated by Carla Marino
ISBN 978 1 84310 657 9
Asperger Syndrome: After the Diagnosis series

Fathering Your Special Child
A Book for Fathers or Carers of Children Diagnosed with Asperger Syndrome
Josie Santomauro
Illustrated by Carla Marino
ISBN 978 1 84310 658 6
Asperger Syndrome: After the Diagnosis series

Your Special Grandchild
A Book for Grandparents of Children Diagnosed with Asperger Syndrome
Josie Santomauro
Illustrated by Carla Marino
ISBN 978 1 84310 659 3
Asperger Syndrome: After the Diagnosis series

Your Special Student
A Book for Educators of Children Diagnosed with Asperger Syndrome
Josie Santomauro and Margaret-Anne Carter
Illustrated by Carla Marino
ISBN 978 1 84310 660 9
Asperger Syndrome: After the Diagnosis series

Your Special Friend
A Book for Peers of Children Diagnosed with Asperger Syndrome
Josie Santomauro
Illustrated by Carla Marino
ISBN 978 1 84310 661 6
Asperger Syndrome: After the Diagnosis series

You Are Special Too

A Book for Brothers and Sisters
of Children Diagnosed
with Asperger Syndrome

JOSIE SANTOMAURO

Illustrated by Carla Marino

Jessica Kingsley *Publishers*
London and Philadelphia

First published in 2009
by Jessica Kingsley Publishers
116 Pentonville Road
London N1 9JB, UK

and

400 Market Street, Suite 400
Philadelphia, PA 19106, USA

www.jkp.com

Copyright © Josie Santomauro 2009
Illustrations copyright © Carla Marino 2009
Printed digitally since 2011

Library of Congress Cataloging in Publication Data
Santomauro, J. (Josie)
    You are special, too : a book for brothers and sisters of children diagnosed with Asperger
syndrome / Josie Santomauro ; illustrated by Carla Marino.
       p. cm.
       ISBN 978-1-84310-656-2 (pb : alk. paper) 1. Asperger's syndrome in
children--Juvenile literature. 2. Asperger's syndrome in children--Patients--Family relation-
ships--Juvenile literature. 3. Brothers and sisters of people with disabilities--Juvenile literature.
I. Title.
    RJ506.A9S3665 2009
    618.92'858832--dc22

                                                          2008042278

British Library Cataloguing in Publication Data
A CIP catalogue record for this book is available from the British Library

ISBN 978 1 84310 656 2
eISBN 978 1 84642 929 3

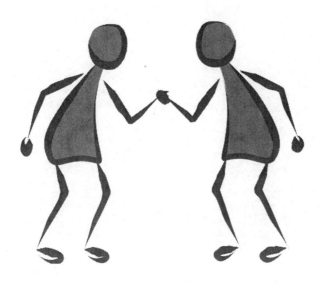

To Chiara
A very special sister

Thank you to all the wonderful
contributors who have given
permission to reprint their gifts of
poetry, reflections, writings and
private thoughts here in this
book.

Contents

What's a Sibling?

First of all, let's see what the word *sibling* means.

The dictionary says:
Sibling = one of two or more children having one or both parents in common.

In 'kid speak' this means a brother or sister.
    So you are a sibling and your brother or sister is a sibling too.

- Does your sibling get special help at school? Like from a teaching assistant?

- They might even go to special classes, or to special teachers, e.g. a speech therapist.

- Your sibling might even go to a special school to learn how to behave appropriately in class.

- Why do you think your sibling needs all this help?

Let's find out why.

Your sibling might be a little different from other kids but they are *not stupid!*

What's Wrong
with My Sibling?

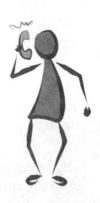

Your sibling needs extra help in four areas:

1. Social skills
2. Communication
3. Behaviour
4. Sensory stimulation.

When somebody needs help so they can function more easily in the community, they may have a disability.

Look at these different types of help others need:

- a person who needs a wheelchair to move around
- a person who needs glasses to see
- a person who needs a puffer for asthma
- a person who needs to use a cane to walk
- a person who needs help to speak clearly
- a person who needs a hearing aid to hear.

Asperger Syndrome?

When you add up these four areas:

1. needs help with people and social skills
2. needs help with talking and communicating with people
3. needs help with behaviour choices
4. needs help with sensory stimulation, as they can find bright lights or noise, for example, very stressful

they equal a disability called *Asperger Syndrome.*

Asperger Syndrome might make life seem a little hard for your sibling

but

Asperger Syndrome also makes your brother or sister special in his or her own way.

Because you are a caring and understanding sibling...

You are special too!

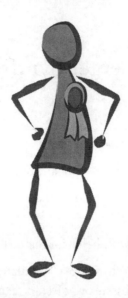

Do you know anyone else who has a sibling with Asperger Syndrome?

Write the names of other special brothers and sisters like you below:

. . . .

. . . .

. . . .

. . . .

. . . .

Introducing
Asperger Syndrome

A nger and frustration

S tress and anxiety

P roblems with speech and language

E asily distracted

R eality/Fiction confusion

G ross motor skills

E ccentric or odd behaviours

R igid and doesn't like change

S ocial skills

Y our sibling can be quite intelligent

N o eye contact

D oesn't like loud noises and crowds

R ote memory

O bsessional

M aking friends is hard

E mpathy

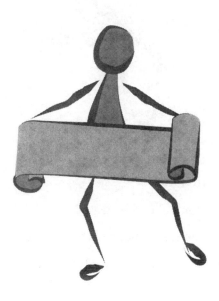

Let's Take a Closer Look at Asperger Syndrome

Anger and frustration

- Your sibling may have temper tantrums when they are angry.

- They might find it hard to ask for help when feeling confused or frustrated.

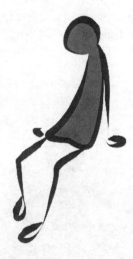

Stress and anxiety

- They don't like to be teased.

- They can sometimes get anxious over changes.

- They can sometimes get stressed at school.

- They need help to learn how to relax and keep calm.

- They need help to ignore teasing and bullying.

Problems with speech and language

- Sometimes they don't realize that their voice is too loud.

- They may have an unusual voice.

- Sometimes they can't explain what they want to say.

- Sometimes they don't understand what people are telling them.

Easily distracted

- Maybe their room and school desk is always untidy.

- Sometimes they forget what someone said to them.

- Sometimes it's hard for them to pay attention, especially in a busy classroom.

Reality/Fiction confusion

- Sometimes they don't understand jokes or stories.

- They might believe that their dreams are real.

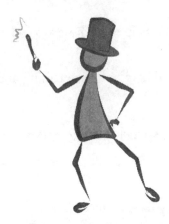

- They get confused if people say things like 'Pull your socks up'.

Gross motor skills

- Sometimes they can be clumsy.
- They might find some sports (especially ball games) a little hard to play.

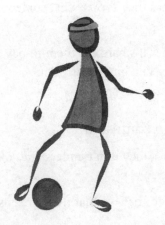

Eccentric or odd behaviours

- They may have different behaviours to other kids.
- Other kids might think they're a bit weird.
- They might do everyday things differently to everyone else.

Rigid and doesn't like change

- They like it better when things don't change.
- They really like things to stay the same.
- They like to know what is going to happen next.

Social skills

- They might find it hard to understand people's body language, like if someone's bored when they're talking.
- They like to talk about their hobbies all the time.
- They may not understand social 'rules' and can sometimes seem rude.

Your sibling can be quite intelligent

- They may be very intelligent – especially at maths, science and computers, and you probably are too!

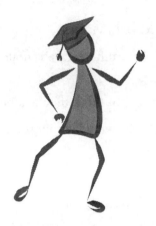

- Some doctors call them 'little professor'.
- They may even go to university when they grow up.

No eye contact

- They don't like to look at people's eyes when they talk to them.
- They might look at the ground instead of someone's face, but they are still listening to them.

Doesn't like loud noises and crowds

- Loud noises can hurt their ears, and bright light may hurt their eyes.

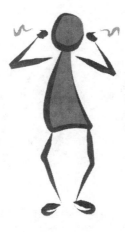

- They don't like noisy or crowded places, like shopping centres or parties.

Rote memory

- They might remember things that happened a long time ago.
- They have a good memory for facts and figures.

Obsessional

- If they really like one or two things they can talk on and on…and on…about it.
- They can do or say something over and over, like flapping their hands, touching their face, or repeating a word.

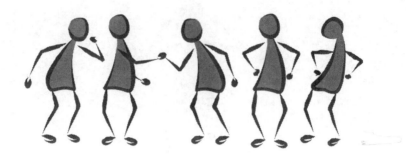

Making friends is hard

- They might not have a lot of friends.

- They might like to have more friends.

- They might not be interested in friends.

- They sometimes find it hard to make new friends.

Empathy

- Sometimes they can't understand how other people are feeling – like if someone is happy or sad.

But here are some other features of Asperger Syndrome:

A rtistic	**S** ignificant
S mart	**Y** why? Asks lots of questions
P unctual	**N** atural
E ngaging	**D** etermined
R epetitive movements	**R** esourceful
G ood natured	**O** ver sensitive
E xtraordinary	**M** aths wiz
R ules	**E** motional

Why Has Your Sibling Got Asperger Syndrome?

How did they get Asperger Syndrome?

- They didn't catch it like when you catch a cold or the chicken pox.

- It's not their fault or your parents' – it's nobody's fault!

- They were probably born like that – but nobody knew until they grew up a bit.

- There is no special cure or magic potion to fix Asperger Syndrome.

- Doctors think a small part of their brain is working differently to other people's.

And *they're not the only one!*

At least one in every 150 people in the world has Asperger Syndrome.

How to Learn More about Asperger Syndrome

Attend a siblings support group meeting.

Join the local Asperger Syndrome support group with your family.

Chat on the internet with other siblings.

Talk to your parents.

Read books about Asperger Syndrome.

Talk to your sibling.

You're Special Too

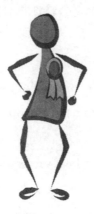

Make yourself a certificate by writing in the most special thing about you, and then present it to yourself!

I . . . .

give myself this certificate because

. . . .

. . . .

. . . .

Presented to myself on __ / __ / __

Signed . . . .

How Can You
Help Your Sibling?

Just by learning to help your sibling you are:

- helping them to have a happy life

and

- helping them to be a successful citizen.

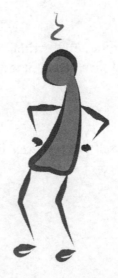

Time out

- If you notice your sibling becoming really stressed at home or at school, you can remind them to take themselves to time out.

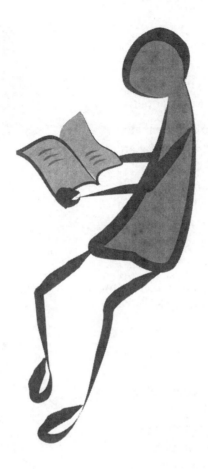

Diary

- Remind them to look at their school diary every day.

- Remind them to write in the dates of any changes or new things that are going to happen, like birthdays or lessons.

Change

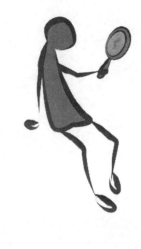

- Warn your sibling about changes they don't know about.

- Try to tell them all about where you are going or what is about to happen. This will make them feel better about what is going to happen.

- Even draw a picture for them, or write down what you know.

Positive

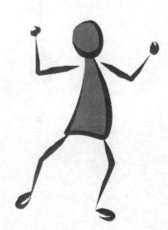

- When your sibling is feeling sad, think of things they like to do and play their favourite game with them.

- Laugh and have fun with them.

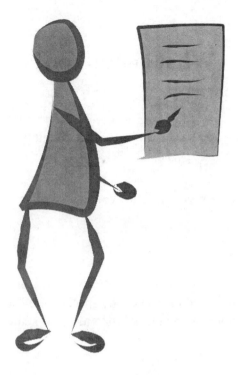

Charts

- Remind them to look at their charts and timetables.

- You can even help them make their own charts.

- Perhaps you might even like to make some charts of your own!

What about You?

Just because you have a sibling with a disability, that doesn't mean you're not special.

Here are some suggestions for you:

Talk

• Talk to your mum, dad or your carer, or even your grandma; somebody special who listens to you when you feel a little sad or even angry.

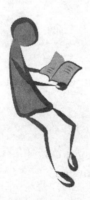

Journal

• Keep a journal or a diary at home for yourself.
• Write in it your thoughts and feelings.
• Try to write in it every day.

Positive

- When you're feeling sad, do something that makes you feel good, like playing with your pet or reading a story.

- Laugh and have fun.

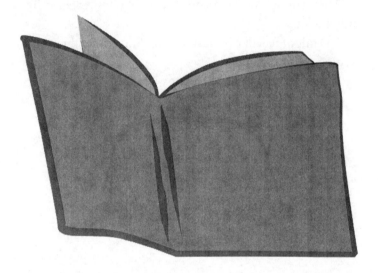

Dial-a-smile

- Collect pictures from magazines, cartoons, photos and drawings that you like and paste them into a scrapbook.

- Feel like relaxing? Or need to be cheered up? Have a look at your Dial-a-smile book!

Mixed Feelings

Sometimes you might feel like you hate your sibling.

They annoy you, and sometimes they're treated differently to you.

You might feel like it's just not fair! Sometimes they might even be embarrassing!

It's ok for you to have feelings like this.

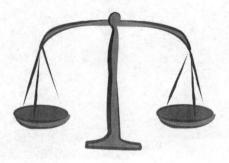

Label the left side of the weighing scales 'Dislikes' and the other 'Likes'.

On the 'Dislikes' side write the things you find annoying about your sibling.

Most of the time you love your sibling. They might be funny and smart. Write on the 'Likes' side of the scales all the things you like about your sibling.

Discover what happens to the scales...

Always remember:

Your love for your sibling will always outweigh the Dislikes!

Write an Acrostic Using Your Name

An acrostic is a series of words where the first letters of each line spell out another word or phrase.

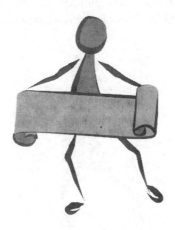

Use special words about you.

For example, if your name is Sam:

S uper

A rtistic

M usician

Remember everybody has a disability of some kind,
It might be big or small.
They might need lots of help
Or none at all.
A disability might be if someone can't swim, can't read,
Needs help with maths or even if they have a big mole
On their nose!
You might even have a disability of some kind.
We're all individuals in this world.
Nobody is perfect!
(Not even the Prime Minister or the President!)
Shhh!! Don't tell them I said that!

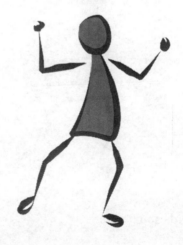

Visit Josie's website: www.booksbyjosie.com.au

Lightning Source UK Ltd.
Milton Keynes UK
UKOW032216131212

203635UK00002B/15/P